TRAINING YOUR OWN SEI

THE COMPLETE GUIDE

SERIES

WORKBOOK

Volume II

Second Edition

Megan Brooks CDT

Imprint: Independently published

All proceeds from this book and other books in this series go directly into funding our service dog training programs.

Thank you for helping make it possible.

Also By This Author:

❖ **Your Dog Wants You to Know The Truth About Commercial Pet Food**

Training your own Service Dog: The Complete Guide Series:
 ❖ -Volume I
 ❖ -Volume III Raising A Service Dog Puppy

Coming Soon:
 ❖ -Training your own Service Dog: The Complete Guide Series Volume IV: Advanced Obedience and Task Training

 ❖ -No Dogs Allowed: A guide to ADA Law for Employers and Business Owners

 ❖ -Know the Law; know your Rights: A guide to ADA law for service dog handlers

MEGA LEARNING METHOD

M otivated

E ffective

G entle

A pproach

L ife Rewards

E arn

A ccelerated

R esults

N ow

I ntensive

N o- nonsense

G oals

Congratulations on deciding to embark on a wonderful journey as you bond with your best friend and partner.

This workbook is designed to be used in conjunction with any and/or all of the books in the Training Your Own Service Dog Series.

Reading Volume I prior to or during using this workbook is extremely important.

Use this training journal to document your training progress over a 28 day period (or longer if you or your dog needs more time or practice).

Daily journal entries are part of the training process where we discuss training goals, procedures; discover what is working and what is not, as well as other insight into your individual training.

Your program

In this workbook, you may choose to work straight through and complete each day's assignment on schedule; however it is not necessary to move that quickly.

Training your own service dog is a lot of work and it is not something you want to rush through. As long as you continue to work daily on material you have already introduced to your dog, you can set your individual program schedule for as short or as long as you would like.

Keep in mind that the first 21 days of the program are extremely intensive. Each of those 21 days a new command is introduced and each day you review the commands introduced from the previous days before as well! This program is not designed to whiz through in a few weeks.

If service dog training took just 4 weeks, everyone would have a service dog that needs one.

I designed the workbook to outline 28 days but I do not, by any means, expect for most of you to actually complete the entire program in 28 consecutive days.

In fact, if you did complete it in 28 consecutive days it is likely the training would not be nearly as solid or reliable as it would be if you set a schedule based on your pace and worked hard rather than fast.

Once the basics are introduced, it will no longer be necessary to do structured training sessions multiple times daily as you must do during the first 28 days or until you have completed the entire workbook. This is providing you are motivated enough to find each and every opportunity to incorporate training into your daily life.

The program consists of one new command introduced per day, after reviewing commands already taught in previous sessions. Make a realistic goal for your timeline on how long it will take to complete the workbook program. No matter for how long in the future you decide to set your individual training goals, I do recommend you find time for at least 2-3 short structured training sessions per day.

By short, I mean 5 minutes or less for young puppies and maybe 10 minutes for adult dogs. You will want to stop the training session while your dog is still interested. Keep them wanting more! Stop before the dog gets tired, bored, full or distracted. Your dog will love the time spent training together and be eager for more.

A note on using punishment in training:

The American Veterinary Society of Animal Behavior (AVSAB) published their position on the use of "punishment" in animal training.

I have covered the four elements of operant conditioning multiple times in each of the books in the series; however I am going to cover this critical information again.

As an owner/trainer of your own service dog, it is very important that you understand the potential adverse effects that are possible when choosing to use certain elements (primarily positive punishment).

People in general tend to think that "punishment" refers to what is actually either "Positive punishment" (+P) and/or "Negative reinforcement" (−R). The reason for this is likely because these elements may use aversives, coercion, physical corrections or even force. In the case of operant conditioning, "positive" does not necessarily mean good or "negative" bad.

Positive simply means the addition of and negative means the removal of.

Whether an element is punishment or reinforcement depends on the goal. Punishment is used to stop a particular behavior while reinforcement encourages (reinforces) a behavior.

+R (Positive Reinforcement) Adds something the subject wants when subject offers desirable behavior = increases desired behavior.

-R (Negative Reinforcement) Removing something unpleasant when subject offers desirable behavior =increases desired behavior.

+P (Positive Punishment) Adding something the subject dislikes when subject offers undesirable behavior = decreases desired behavior.

-P (Negative Punishment) Removing something the subject wants when subject offers undesirable behavior = decreases desired behavior.

Veterinary behaviorists and other animal behaviorists most commonly use a combination of positive reinforcement and negative punishment. I also choose to use these two elements as my primary strategies and recommend that you do as well.

When you choose a professional trainer to oversee the training of your service dog, I highly recommend that you find a trainer who abides by these guidelines and avoid trainers who train using outdated methods (known as traditional training).

When you are screening trainers, ask questions. Some trainers will tell you that they use positive training methods but they also employ traditional elements as well.

Any trainer who uses training collars such as a choke chain or prong/pinch collars is a traditional trainer. If a trainer focuses too much on "dominance" and uses methods such as the Alpha Roll, this is also outdated training methods and should not be your chosen trainer. Another clue is trainers who use the old methods rarely train with clickers.

There are many reasons why +P is ineffective and even more concerning is the potential negative effects that can result from this element of training.

First, it must be understood that a behavior exists because at some point it has been (or continues to be) unintentially reinforced in some way.

Even the fact that you cannot punish an unwanted behavior consistently each time it occurs if you are not there to see it every single time can reinforce the behavior simply by putting the self- reward an animal gets from this behavior on a random reinforcement schedule (proven to STRENGTHEN a behavior).

Other reasons that the AVSAB advises against using positive punishment (at least) as the first response to an unwanted behavior include:

1. It is difficult to time correctly and timing is crucial in training.
2. The intensity must be strong enough the FIRST time for it to be effective.
3. If the intensity is not strong enough, the behavior will not stop and instead the animal may essentially get used to the correction (known as habituation).
4. If the intensity of a positive punishment is too strong or is done out of anger or frustration it can actually cause physical harm.
5. It can cause intense fear and/or aggression.
6. It can suppress warnings of an impending bite if an animal has been punished for growling.
7. It can lead to negative associations with the person delivering the punishment.
8. It does not teach the appropriate behavior.

Instead of using positive punishment methods, unless adequate attempts have been made to use all other options first, it is important to focus on REINFORCING the desired behavior you would rather be performed in its place as well as identifying and removing whatever is reinforcing the unwanted behavior by addressing the conditions.

This strategy promotes better understanding of your dog's behavior and better awareness of how we contribute to the behaviors developing in the first place. In addition, it fosters the trust and the bond between you and your dog.

Summary:

Never use positive punishment as a strategy, unless you have already made every possible attempt to correct the behavior using positive reinforcement combined with negative punishment and are aware of the potential dangers and pitfalls of using positive punishment.

Instead, determine what is reinforcing unwanted behavior, remove that reward and reinforce (reward) an alternate behavior that can replace the unwanted behavior.

List Your Goals In Training:

1.

2.

3.

4.

5.

Lesson Day 1:

Reward the behavior you like while preventing, ignoring or interrupting behavior you do not.

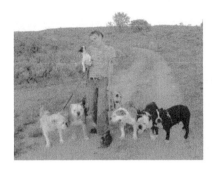

All dogs that come with me are immediately placed on my leadership program.

My program quickly and gently teaches them to always look to me for direction, to respect the order of our "pack" and to feel comfortable that they do not have to worry about anything.

As the pack leader, you will lead them, provide guidance and protect them from danger.

Providing your dog has settled in nicely, (if he or she is a rescue case) they will be eager to begin learning. Dogs LOVE training when you do it in a positive fashion.

I NEVER bully, intimidate or yell at dogs. I do not use metal "choke" chains or prong (pinch) collars. There is no need for it!

Instead I take a positive approach. The concept is so simple….

This teaches all dogs quickly and gently what I expect from them as well as what is unacceptable.

Charging the clicker

I highly recommend using a clicker to teach new behaviors while working this program.

If you choose, you can substitute a sound or a word (such as "Yes!") for 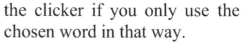 the clicker if you only use the chosen word in that way.

In order for the clicker to work, you must first give it a meaning. We call this "charging" the clicker.

How to charge the clicker

Step 1- Armed with treats and a clicker; begin to click for no apparent reason.

Step 2- Each click earns a reward

Step 3- Watch for the moment your dog looks at you when he hears the click. It is now the dog has made the connection and the clicker is charged.

Date:

Training goal of the day:

Lesson Day 2:

To give a command, one must first have a dog's full attention.

Name/Watch me

Phase I

Right away, we introduce the hand signal that means "look at me and wait for further instruction".

The verbal command is the dog's name and I introduce both the verbal cue and the hand signal simultaneously.

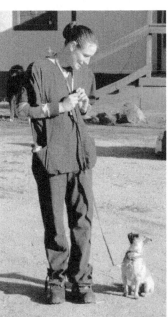

Step 1- Use a food reward or toy (depending on the dog's preference).

Step 2- Wave the lure in front of the dog's face to get their attention.

Step 3- SLOWLY lead their gaze to your face and as soon as they look at you, say their name and reward them using a treat from your pouch (not the lure).

Step 4- Repeat 10 times in a row as many times as possible throughout the day.

Step 5- Continue doing this exercise throughout the entire training program.

**This exercise is crucial in order to train your dog that when you say their name they are to look at you. When this happens, you can be confident you should always be able to get your dog's attention.

Name/Watch me

Phase II

Step 1- Instead of leading your dog's gaze to your face with the treat as you did in *Phase I*, you will hold the treat out to your side in your left hand.

Step 2-Wait for your dog to take his eyes off of the treat and look at you.

Step 3- Ensure you don't miss the split second this occurs so you can "Capture" it with a click and treat.

.

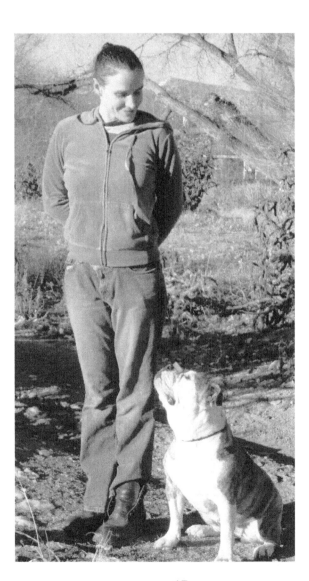

Step 4- Reach into your treat pouch and reward from your right hand.

Date:

Training Goal of the day:

Lesson Day 3:

Use a Marker

What is the Clicker/Marker?

Karen Pryor, a marine mammal trainer, first introduced clicker training to dog training in the late 80's.

The clicker is a training tool that, when pressed, makes a distinct click. The click clarifies in the dog's mind that whatever he or she was doing at the time the click was delivered is the correct thing to do.

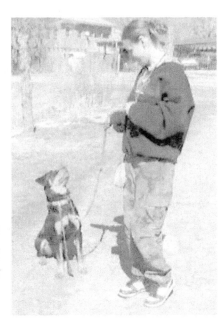

The clicker, after being "charged" or "conditioned", is a message to the dog that a reward was earned. When used during the initial phases of training, learning comes quickly.

Marker or Clicker training is based on two scientific principles: classical conditioning and operant conditioning.

**Remember: You have 1 second to mark a behavior as correct, and then your dog moves on to the next moment. A late click rewards the wrong behavior.

SIT

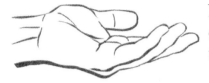 Next is the hand signal for "Sit". Most dogs catch onto "Sit" very quickly. Again, I begin training silently using a lure.

Step 1- Place food in contact with nose.

Step 2- Raise food over dog's head and back towards the forehead (Not too high or your dog will jump up).

Step 3- Dog looks up and folds into a sit position.

Step 4- Click and treat.

Step 5- Repeat

After just a few repetitions, most dogs are eagerly sitting for the reward. Once the dog "gets it" I will begin to add the verbal cue

**Since we are not yet teaching "Stay" I do not correct the dog for getting up, but instead use it as an opportunity to do another repetition.

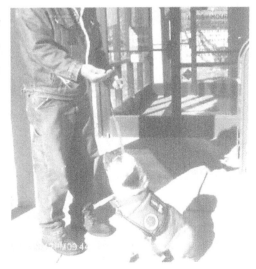

Date:

Training goal of the day:

Lesson Day 4:

Just be quiet at first

Begin training silently using a lure.

The food lure eventually becomes the hand signal for a given behavior.

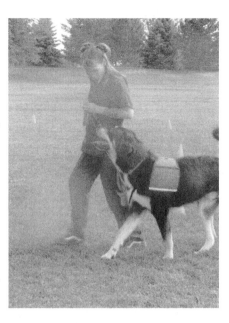

Try to refrain from chanting the commands this early in training. The dog "gets it" when 9 out of 10 times the dog complies within a few seconds.

Once you achieve 90% accuracy, then you may begin to add the verbal cue. How you add the verbal cue is VERY important!

**AGAIN: Adding the cue generally does not come into practice until the dog is RELIABLY following the hand signal 80-90% of the time.

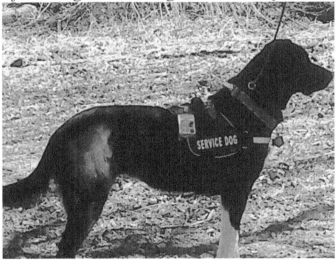

COME

The "Come" command is known as the Recall.

Many dog owners have a great deal of trouble with this one and many dogs have been inadvertently taught NOT to come when called at some point.

Upon coming to me for training, the recall is often a dog's very favorite command of all. I do tons of work on it and practice makes perfect.

Even if you only do 10 repetitions a day, after a month you have 300 repetitions under your team's collar. I recommend many more daily repetitions. There is no such thing as "too many" repetitions of the recall.

Work daily on "recalls" using any opportunity you can possibly find to practice. Do everything from calling them from another room in the house to structured "Stay" and "Come"; first on-leash and gradually building on that.

Perhaps the best practice is calling them when they are running free in a safe area and heartily rewarding them with treats and praise. Add an even more valuable reward by allowing them to go and play again.

Rules:

-Your dog MUST come every time you call them, no matter what! If they choose not to, you must enforce it.

-If it is an issue that they are not coming when called you are giving them too much freedom and must do structured recall practice before allowing such freedom.

**Also, I will never call them if I am not 100 % sure they will come or am in a position to enforce it. If your dog is chasing a squirrel, calling them is only going to damage your training.

Long Line Recall

Step 1- In a place with no distractions; clip a 15-foot leash to your dog's flat-buckle collar.

Step 2- Allow your dog to lose focus on you and wander off, sniff, explore etc.

Step 3-Say your dog's name to get his attention. When he looks at you give the verbal cue and hand signal.

Step 4- When your dog gets to you; give him lots of hearty praise and reward.

Step 5- Reward the highest value reward of all and release your dog to go explore again.

Step 6- Repeat as many times as possible.

**Note: During the first few long-line recalls, your dog likely thinks he is actually off-leash and may challenge your ability to enforce your request.

I included some tips below in case you have any issues such as this.

-Give the verbal cue in a happy excited voice. If necessary, clap your hands and call to your dog in a high-pitched voice.

-Back up a few steps, turn and run the other way or squat down and open your arms out to your sides while calling your dog in the most irresistible way you can imagine.

-Give the end of the line a gentle tug to get your dog moving on his way to you.

-Avoid having to reel your dog to you, try using the other suggestions first to get him to come to you on this own.

-Praise and reward heartily no matter how the dog makes it to you or how long it takes.

-If your dog does not come running to you immediately in celebration, you need to work on many more repetitions of recalls.

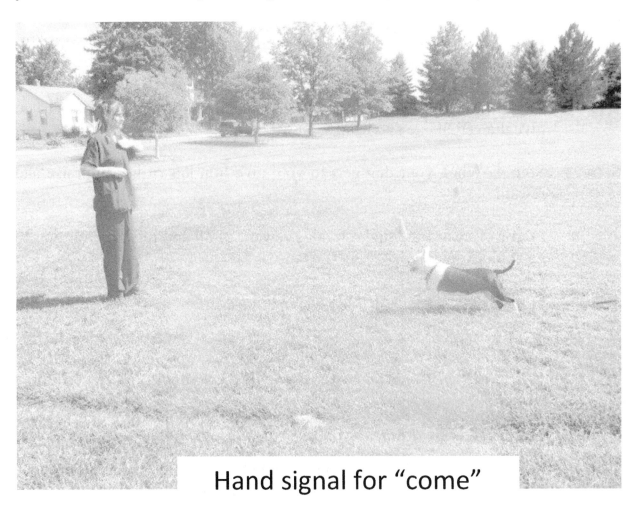

Hand signal for "come"

Date:

Training Goal of the day:

Lesson Day 5:

Achieve big goals by taking baby steps (shaping).

Some dogs take a little longer to get it and I will use a known as "Shaping" where I reward small increments with the goal of eventually accomplishing a finished action.

To teach a "Down" using shaping, I will use my lure and release the reward every time the dog takes a step closer. At first, the butt may pop up each time I lower the lure. When this happens, I say "Uh-oh!" and take the reward away (removal technique).

I will ask for another "Sit" and try again. As soon as I get the dog to lower their head without raising the butt I will reward that.

After several repetitions when I know the dog "gets it" I will up the ante and not reward a simple lowering of the head. Now the dog must figure out what I want.

The next step may be lowering one or both elbows which I reward heartily for a while! Again, once this is mastered I will begin to hold off the reward for a closer approximation.

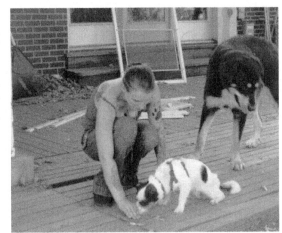

Stay

Once your dog learns the basics of "Sit" and "Down" I begin to teach the very important command "Stay".

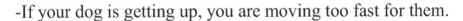

"Stay" is VERY structured and is easy to ruin if you do not teach it carefully.

***"Stay" means to stay right where I left you and ABSOLUTELY do not move until I give you another directive.*

-If your dog is getting up, you are moving too fast for them.

-Practice the "Down-stay" and "Sit-stay" (separately) many times a day in non-distracting situations.

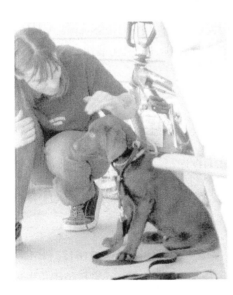

-If your dog breaks the "Stay", you MUST be right there to correct them and put them back in the same spot until given a release command.

If you don't notice the dog broke until even a couple of seconds later, the dog forgot he was even on a "Stay" and also learned that nothing was keeping him there!

Tethered "Stay"

The tethered "Stay", I believe, is very important for any dog to be taught.

If a dog is never taught to hold a tethered stay I have very little faith that any dog would not suffer a certain amount of stress if it became necessary to tie your dog momentarily (one day in an emergency or if you are on vacation and simply want sit in the jacuzzi or get a massage) without worrying about your dog or leaving him behind or in the car.

Begin teaching the tethered "Stay" after you have advanced to *Phase II* of the traditional "Stay".

The dog can be in any position, as long as they are quiet.

**Tip: You may want to use a chain leash or cable tie for this exercise if your dog may chew through your leash when tied to a stationary object.

Step 1- Attach your dog's tie to a flat buckle collar or harness (NEVER tether a dog using a training collar) and attach the tie to a stationary object.

Step 2- Give the verbal cue and hand signal for "stay. Turn and walk about 6-feet away.

Step 3- Stay away only about 5-10 seconds at first.

**Tip: Try and get back to reward and release your dog BEFORE he begins to whine and fuss.

Step 4- If your dog remains quiet, return to your dog to praise and reward. Ignore any fussing and wait for just a few seconds of quiet to return and reward the dog.

Step 5- Gradually add time you can tether your dog and walk 6 feet away while he remains quiet. If he really fusses, do not try and do 10 seconds just yet. Start at 2 or 3 seconds or even only 3 feet away and work from there.

Step 6- Practice daily and move onto phase II only when you can move 6 feet away and your dog can quietly stay tethered for 3 minutes.

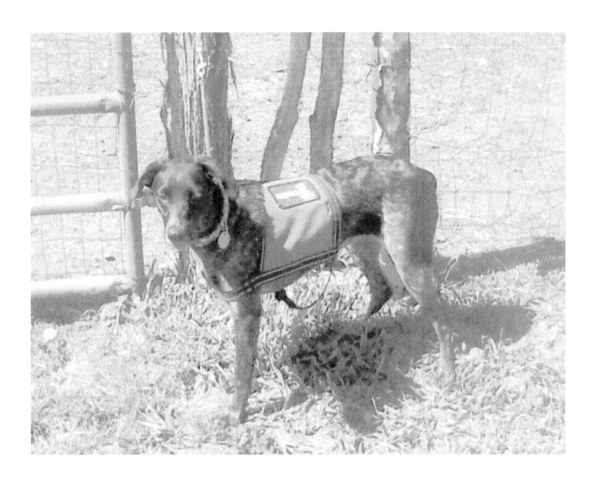

Date:

Training Goal of the day:

Lesson Day 6:

Find what motivates your dog

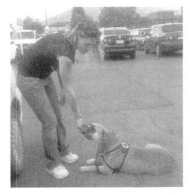 Most dogs are at least partially motivated by food, however, some are not.

Some dogs are most motivated by chasing a ball or a favorite toy. Some dogs, a game of Tug-of-war.

A select number of dogs are motivated simply by your affection.

It is crucial to find what it is that motivates your particular dog.

If you are desperately trying to train using cheese tidbits and your dog is simply not interested, you are selling yourself short on opportunities for training.

Experiment and find what does work for your particular dog.

What foods are high-value to your dog?

What toys?

Games?

A belly rub and a "good boy"?

Loose-Leash Walking

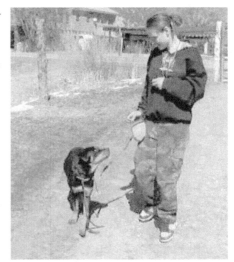

My rule of thumb is the leash MUST always be loose! The leash should ONLY ever become tight for a split second to give the dog feedback that he needs to pay closer attention.

There are many methods of teaching loose leash walking.

The method I use is a method I developed myself and if used correctly almost always works in 10 minutes or less.

I use a training collar rather than clipping the leash to the flat buckle collar. The training collar I use is called a slip collar and it is made of nylon. Picture a show lead. It works the way a "choke chain" is supposed to work but it is much more effective and much safer.

Step 1- Keeping your leash short but always loose, and with the training collar high on the neck behind the ears and your arm at your side, start walking. You can almost always anticipate that the dog will forge ahead.

Step 2- BEFORE the leash becomes tight, stop in your tracks, then immediately change directions and head in the opposite direction at a fast pace.

Step 3- Continue changing directions, keeping it unpredictable so your dog learns quickly to pay attention to where you are at.

Note: It is the suddenness of hitting the end of the leash, not the force that is effective.

Tips:

-Stay happy and upbeat during this exercise, especially when you change directions.

-Do not forget to praise and reward heartily when your dog is in the correct position.

-Treat next to your pant seam where you want your dog's head to be, she will start spending more and more time there.

Date:

Training Goal of the day:

Lesson Day 7:

Teach impulse control

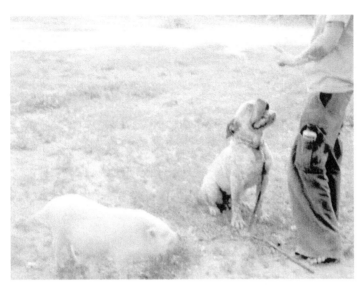 While I am teaching the commands "Name", "Sit", "Down" etc. we are also working on other things.

Impulse control is critical for your service dog to learn so the "Wait" command is one of the very first cues I teach.

"Wait" is VERY important for any dog but especially for your service dog. "Wait" is much less structured than the formal "Stay" command.

"Wait" simply teaches your dog to control his natural impulsiveness. It literally means "Wait for me to give you permission to proceed or another command".

I usually ask dogs to "Wait" when they are in a sitting position because they are more likely to "Wait" if they are focused on sitting. I may ask a dog to "Wait" dozens of times a day! I ask them to "Wait" for anything that they may deem pleasurable.

I ask them to "Wait" before meals; treats; playing a game; being given a toy; going for a walk; jumping in our out of the car; and even before going outside and coming inside.

Date:

Training Goal of the day:

Training Activity:

Restrained Recall

Object: This exercise teaches a prompt recall and strengthens your dog's desire to come to you when called by way of exploiting his pack drive just a tad.
Prerequisites: None
Difficulty: Easy
Items needed: You will need a 15-foot long line, some treats and a partner for this exercise.

Step 1- Have your partner hold your dog while you walk away from the dog, about 15 or 20-feet. Your partner should not engage with dog but should hold the leash fairly short so the dog has to strain to try and follow you (likely this will happen before you even call the dog).

Step 2- Allow the dog to get a bit worked up and frustrated. This is what makes the exercise so effective. No need to wait for the dog to stop fussing for this exercise.

Step 3- Call your dog to you and when your dog is straining hard in an

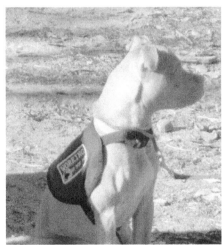 attempt to come to you your partner releases the dog.

This week I feel proud of my team because:

We need improvement in these areas:

Week 1 Notes:

Lesson Day 8:

Timing is critical

Your dog associates a behavior with a consequence (positive or negative) in just 1 second. This means the saying "You have to catch them in the act" is critically true.

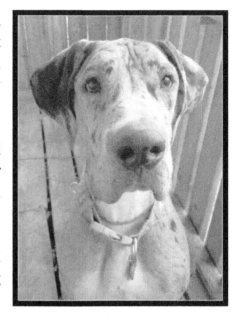

To correct a dog for an unwanted behavior even two or three seconds after the fact is meaningless to the dog and damaging to your training.

A dog believes they are being corrected or rewarded for whatever they are doing at THAT EXACT moment.

Timing means you must watch your dog closely enough that you see mistakes or triumphs exactly when they occur so you can either reward or correct them instantly. Dogs live completely in the present.

Down

I begin teaching dogs the "Down" command from as sitting position.

I use my lure, which can be anything the dog may enjoy. I lure their face slowly to the floor with the treat.

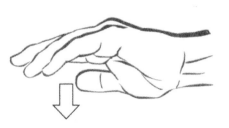

Many dogs will go right into a "Down" position as they try to get the reward.

When this happens, if I am at the point of adding the verbal cue I say "Down!" as soon as they lie down, release the reward.

Step 1- Begin in a "Sit" position.

Step 2- Lure dog's nose to floor with a nibble of food.

Step 3- Click and treat when dog goes all the way down

***Troubleshooting: If your dog's rear pops up, say "Uh-oh!" and remove the treat. Start over by asking for a "sit" and resume luring the dog down from a "sit" position. Repeat as necessary.*

Date:

Training Goal of the day:

Lesson Day 9:

Just because the door is open does not mean that you have permission to go through it.

1. Sit at the door
2. Sit while I reach 4 inches toward the knob
3. Sit while I reach 8 inches toward the knob
4. Sit while I touch the knob
5. Sit while I jiggle the knob
6. Sit while I open the door a crack
7. Sit while I open the door 2 inches
8. Sit while I open the door 5 inches
9. Sit while I open the door 1 foot
10. Sit while I open the door 2 feet
11. Sit while I open the door 4 feet
12. Sit while I take 1 step into the open doorway
13. Sit while I take 2 steps into the open doorway
14. Sit while I walk all the way through the doorway and turn around

If your dog gets up at any step, say "Uh-oh!" and close the door. If she breaks again, go back to previous step.

Any time you say "Uh-oh!" three times in a row, you have taken too big of a step between behaviors. Go back to the previous step.

Wait

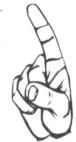

Step 1-Set your dog up in normal, everyday situations where he would normally take it upon himself to bolt through the door or gobble up the turkey you just dropped on the floor.

Step 2- As soon as your dog goes to move forward, physically block him and tell him "Wait".
I use my index finger as the hand signal.

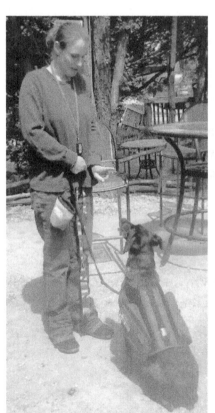

Step 3- Back up just enough to give him an opportunity to try to go for it again. When he goes to make a move, physically block him again and using the hand signal, repeat the command "Wait".

Step 4- Once he surrenders to your "Wait" command, release him by stepping way back and giving an upbeat "OK!"!

Step 5- Practice several times daily in any situation where this command could be of use.

Date:

Training Goal of the day:

Lesson Day 10:

Go pee.

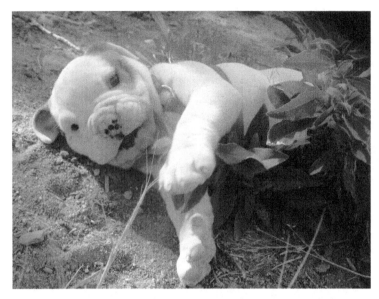

It is essential for service dogs to learn how to go on cue. You can choose any word you feel comfortable with.

**At home, it really helps to always take them to the same place where you want your dog to eliminate. Doing this not only helps the dog learn faster but* also makes yard duty much less of a chore!*

This is very simple. Take them outside to the spot frequently and "capture" the behavior of elimination by labeling it (giving the verbal cue right as they are doing it).

Before long, you can give the cue and they will do their duty!

**Capture- training method in which you wait for a behavior to occur so you can reward it and put it on cue.*

Date:

Training Goal of the day:

Lesson Day 11:

Consistency is the key.

Consistency is indeed the key!

If each person in your household has different rules and expectations for the dog, he would end up extremely confused and likely pretty naughty as well.

Everyone in your household must decide on the rules and stick to them.

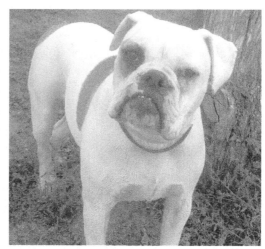

There is no gray area for dogs. Your training always must be very clear. A rule is a rule.

**For example, if you want your dog to sit before being petted, you must consistently reinforce this.*

- ❖ You must be clear in your training.
- ❖ You must be 100% consistent. This will produce a dog that feels safe and trusting.

Targeting

Targeting is the act of teaching your dog to touch a target with his nose, paw or both. Eventually this translates into asking your dog to do tasks such as switching the lights on or off or using his paw to use the automatic handicap accessible door.

Paw
Method 1:

Step 1- Armed with treats and a clicker, sit on the floor facing your dog in a sitting position.

Step 2- Pick up your dog's paw as you click, treat and repeat.

Step 3- Keep at it! Your dog will eventually make the connection and lift up his own paw. When he does this, give him a jackpot of treats and lots of praise.

Don't worry if he doesn't get it again for a while, he will.

Method 2:

Step 1- With your dog in a sitting position, use a treat and hold it just above his nose. Move the treat slightly towards the back of his body and over his head so he has to lift his front paws off the ground to reach it.

Step 2- When your dog's paw or paws leave the ground, touch one.

Step 3- Click, treat and repeat.

Nose/Touch

In this case we will use your first two fingers.

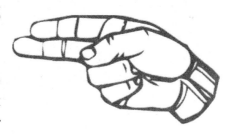

I like to use a sticker stuck on my two outstretched fingers as the target so that later on I can move the sticker wherever I want him to "Touch".

Step 1- With a treat in your palm, hold out your two outstretched fingers and wait for your dog to touch it with his nose. This shouldn't take long because dogs explore everything with their noses. Make sure to capture the moment by clicking at the exact moment and releasing the treat.

Step 2- Soon your dog will figure out that what you want is for him to touch the target with his nose. When this happens you can begin to add the verbal cue "Touch".

Step 3- Start moving the target around so your dog has to follow it in order to touch it.

Target stick

Teach targeting using a target stick for either paw or nose. Any stick will work.

Step 1-Put a dab of peanut butter on the end and click when your dog licks the peanut butter (the peanut butter is the treat).

Step 2- Start moving the target stick around in different places and reward when your dog touches it.

Or for paw:

Step 1-Touch the dog's paw with the stick.

Step 2- Click, treat and repeat.

Step 3-Hold stick near dog's paw until he learns to touch it himself Start moving the target stick around, touching different places and reward when your dog touches it.

Laser pointer:

Step 1- Point laser light at food or a favorite toy.

Step 2- As dog learns to touch laser dot, begin moving the laser dot around to different places.

Step 3- Click, treat and repeat.

**Be very careful not to shine laser light into a dog's eyes.

Date:

Training Goal of the day:

Lesson Day 12:

Avoid repeating commands.

One of the biggest mistakes many of my clients (and likely any human) makes is repeating the cue, in this case "Sit", over and over when the dog is standing, sniffing or running away.

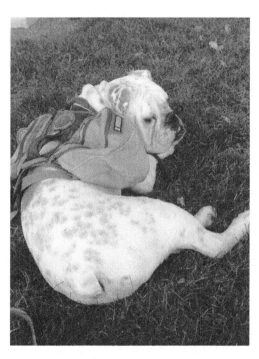

Chanting commands at your dog that he does not understand is inadvertently teaching your dog to ignore you! Remember, dogs do not speak English (or Spanish, Northern Tiwa, German, French etc.)

You must teach them what these words mean. My strategy is to label the word for them. To label the word in any command, you simply say the command clearly just as they comply with the task.

For example, for "Sit" I use my hand signal and as soon as they plop into the "Sit" position I say "Sit!!"

Of course lots of praise and reward goes into each successful "Sit" at this point in training.

Heel

Equally, if not more important than the other commands I introduce in the first week is the "Heel" command.

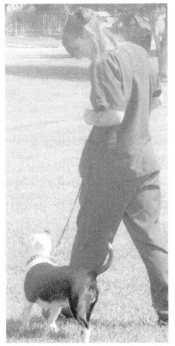

Dogs are traditionally trained to work on the handler's left side, but you can train your service dog on whichever side is most comfortable for you.

You and your dog are now partners and this is demonstrated as you walk. If your dog were to be in front of you, he or she would be assuming the leadership role by default. When this happens, you lose authority in the partnership.

Therefore it is crucial your dog walk beside you at least any time the dog is working. I communicate this clearly on day one and most dogs are glad to learn a more comfortable way to take walks rather than choking themselves!

**To begin to teach "Heel", you should have already mastered the loose leash walk.*

To hold the leash properly, hook the loop over your thumb. Gather and hold the slack from the top half of the leash in the same hand.

**I tie a knot about halfway down a 4-foot leash as a guide. I never hold the leash any tighter than the knot and the*

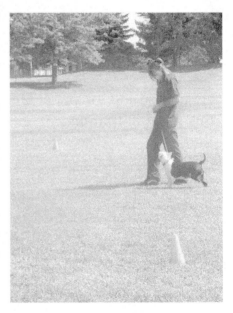

knot helps me hold onto the leash more securely.

Leave only enough slack so there is no tension felt on the leash between you and the dog. There should always be a "U" in the leash where the snap clips onto the collar.

Step 1- Begin with the dog sitting in the "Heel" position.

Step 2- Make eye contact and in a happy voice say "Name, Heel!" and step off with the foot closest to your dog.

Step 3- Label "Heel" as you walk when your dog is in the "Heel" position.

Step 4- Praise and reward, treating at your pant seam.

Step 5- To stop, halt forward movement with the foot farthest from the dog and bring the closest leg up to meet it. (The foot closest to dog is the last to move). As you plant the last foot, cue or lure "Sit".

Step 6- Praise and reward

Tips:
-Begin with just one or two steps and then halt/cue "Sit".

-Any time there is pressure on the leash; stop and cue "Sit" or change directions.

-Do not just walk in a straight line. Teach your dog to follow you through turns and direction changes. Halt and cue "Sit" often.

-Practice pylon heeling exercises often.

-As your dog improves, add other obedience cues (Down, Sit or Down-stay, Recall etc.).

-At halt, walk all the way around your dog while he stays sitting.

-Be creative in how you vary training.

-Always praise returning to heel position.

-Never allow the leash to become tight. It must be loose to communicate feedback and the more you pull the more your dog will pull (opposition defiance reflex).

- Add distractions from low to moderate.

-Apply leash pressure for only an instant and immediately release.

-Practice turning towards your dog and away from your dog (about turns).

Add pace changes
1. Normal pace
2. Change to slow pace
3. Normal pace
4. Change to fast pace
5. Normal pace

Date:

Training Goal of the day:

Lesson Day 13:

Map it out

Always have a mental picture of how a finished behavior will look and how you plan to achieve it.

Once you have an idea of how the finished behavior will look, map out your training plan in steps.
How does the finished behavior look? What steps are you going to take to get there?

**Example: Teaching a seizure response dog to bring a phone and a blanket to the partner at the onset of a seizure, and then lie beside handler until help arrives or seizure subsides.*

The response behavior is cued (triggered) by the handler slumping down.

-What does this look like?

-What methods will go into training this sequence and in what order?

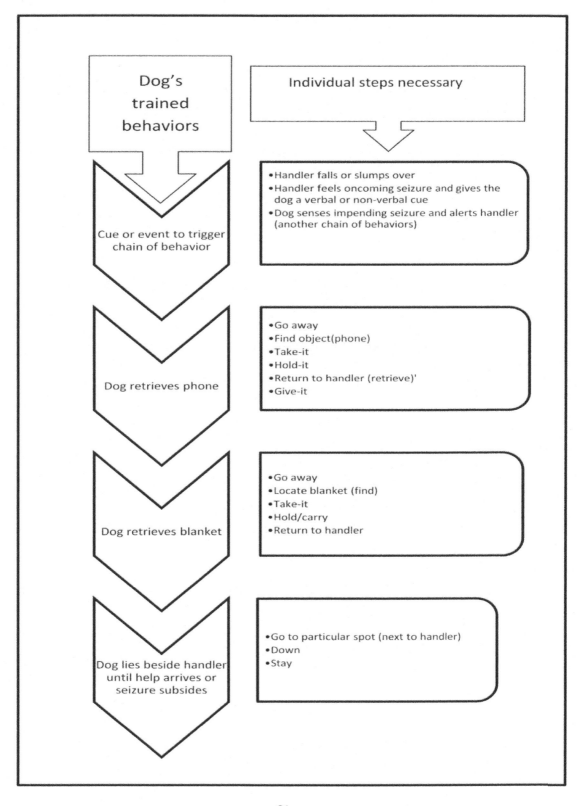

Dog's trained behaviors	Individual steps necessary
Cue or event to trigger chain of behavior	• Handler falls or slumps over • Handler feels oncoming seizure and gives the dog a verbal or non-verbal cue • Dog senses impending seizure and alerts handler (another chain of behaviors)
Dog retrieves phone	• Go away • Find object(phone) • Take-it • Hold-it • Return to handler (retrieve)' • Give-it
Dog retrieves blanket	• Go away • Locate blanket (find) • Take-it • Hold/carry • Return to handler
Dog lies beside handler until help arrives or seizure subsides	• Go to particular spot (next to handler) • Down • Stay

Leave it

**Note: Have your dog on-leash when you practice just to avoid her accidentally rewarding herself with the forbidden treat.

Step 1- Place a low value treat or item on the ground, guarding it with your hand if necessary. Say "Leave-it" in a stern and commanding voice. The second the dog looks away from the treat, click, praise and reward using a very high value food reward that your dog will like (Not the item you told him to leave).

Step 2- Practice 10 repetitions per session. Try to have several short sessions during the day when you can.

You are ready for *Phase II* when you no longer have to guard the treat with your hand.

Phase II

Step 1- Place a low value treat or item on the ground and say "Leave-it" in a commanding voice.

Step 2- As soon as she looks at **you**, start to back up and use a high pitched voice if necessary to encourage your dog to leave the item and come to you.

Step 3- As soon as she starts to come, click and reward using a high value food reward. Repeat.

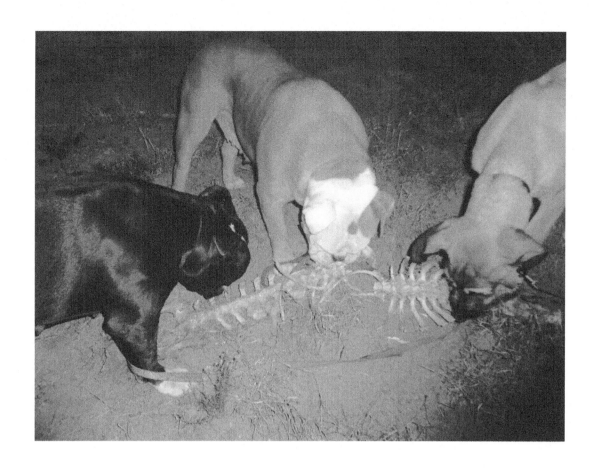

Date:

Training Goal of the day:

Lesson Day 14:

Games make training fun!

Here are links to several training games and brain games for dogs:

https://moderndogmagazine.com/articles/10-socialization-training-games-you-should-play-your-puppy/119978

https://www.mnn.com/family/pets/stories/10-brain-games-to-play-with-your-dog

https://www.wideopenpets.com/10-games-keep-dog-mentally-stimulated/

https://www.whole-dog-journal.com/training/leash_training/games-for-building-reliable-recall-behavior-for-your-dog/

https://journeydogtraining.com/13-dog-training-games/

https://www.canidae.com/blog/2015/11/6-learning-games-to-play-with-your-puppy/

https://mom.com/momlife/17986-beyond-fetch-10-other-games-play-your-dog

http://barkercise.com/boredom-busters-games-for-dogs/

https://mktreattruck.com/dog-games

Date:

Training Goal of the day:

Training Activity:

Pylon Heeling Exercise

Goal: To teach focus and reinforce heeling on leash
Difficulty: Easy
Prerequisites: None
Items needed: 6-8 small soccer cones, leash, clicker and treats

Place the cones (or other objects) 20 feet between 2 rows in a staggered formation (see diagram below) about 15 feet apart, depending on space.

You will weave through the formation with your dog and practice left and right turns. If you have 6 cones you will make three left turns and three right turns each round.

When you weave through the formation, assuming your dog is on your left; one row will practice left turns (into your dog) and the other row, right turns (away from your dog). If you work your dog on the right side, of course, this would be the opposite.

On turns where you turn towards your dog, you will not use treats but do use your opposite knee to bump your dog a little bit as you go in a half circle around the cone until he figures this exercise out.

Your dog's nose must remain in-line with your leg/wheelchair or the pylon exercise doesn't work.

On the row where you turn away from your dog you will use a treat. Hold the treat next to your pant seam or a little behind starting just before you begin the half circle around the cone and lead your dog around with you. Release the treat after you complete going around the cone.

Increase your speed as you and your dog improve.

** For trainers using a wheelchair or other mobility aid, take the turn into your dog the same way as described for non-wheelchair handlers. Essentially you "cut your dog off" before he gets ahead of your chair or walker.

*Again, for handlers using a wheelchair, treat at your wheel right about in-line with your hip.

Pylon Heeling 4 Levels

Level 1- Command every pylon, LOTS of praise between pylons, food reward on OUTSIDE pylons only. If bumping on inside pylon make correction (bump).

Level 2- Same as level 1. No praise between pylons.

Level 3- Command at beginning, no command or reward until 3rd outside pylon.

Level 4- Command at beginning. No rewards or commands until end. If your dog makes a mistake go back to level 1 or 2.

Level 5- Same as level 1 off lead

Level 6- Same as level 2 off lead

Level 7- Same as level 3 off lead

Level 8- Same as level 4 off-lead

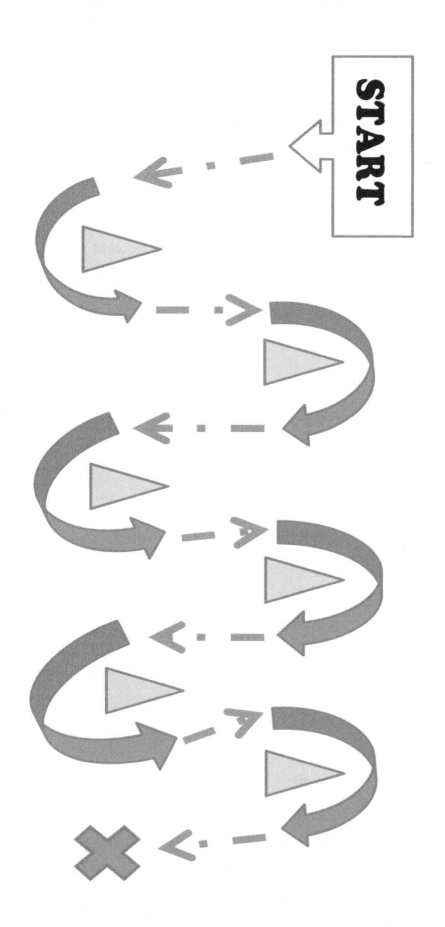

PYLON HEELING EXERCISE

START

This week I feel proud of my team because:

We need improvement in these areas:

Week 2 Notes:

Lesson Day 15:

Never be afraid to go back a step if your dog gets tripped up

It can be incredibly frustrating when suddenly one day your dog seems to have forgotten everything previously learned.

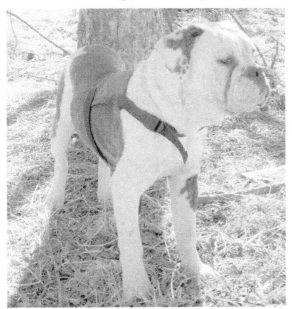

No worries! This is completely normal and easily solved by slowing down a bit. Simply go back a step, to the last place your dog was successful and work there for a bit. When your dog remembers what to do, the trained response will be even more solid.

Stand

With any dog, teaching "Stand" is a useful behavior for grooming and veterinary exams. However a reliably trained "Stand" command is essential for service dogs because it makes it easier to dress them in their uniform for work.

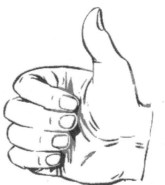

Step 1– Put a food reward in your right hand and hold your dog's leash in the left hand. With your right hand, make a fist with the food tidbit closed inside and your thumb pointing up like the "thumbs up" signal. This becomes the hand signal for "Stand".

Step 2- Stand facing your dog directly in front of them. Ask them to "Sit" or "Down" (train each separately) and "Stay" if you choose.

Step 3- Allow him to smell the treat in your hand so he knows it is there but do not give the "thumbs up" signal until you are ready.

Step 4- Once your dog is sitting (or laying down) and aware of the food reward, simultaneously give the "thumbs up" signal, back up a step or two and use the leash to encourage your dog to stand.

Step 5- As soon as your dog lifts his rear end off of the ground be prepared to click and treat!

Step 6- Repeat 5-10 times per session Remember NOT to add a verbal cue until the command is reliable at around 90%

**Note: You are training a "Stand". You do not want him to take a step once he stands so do not back up too many steps, just enough to give him room.

Date:

Training goal of the day:

Lesson Day 16:

Adding the 3 D's

The Three Ds *proof* behaviors and help ensure they are under *stimulus control*.

A behavior is considered to be under stimulus control when the dog responds consistently to the cue for that behavior and does not offer the behavior unless the cue is given. The 3 D's are duration, distance, and distraction.
All three combined verify mastery of the behavior.

Build a strong foundation before increasing the difficulty of any criteria.

Duration is the length of time the dog sustains the behavior. Just because a dog understands how to "Stay" for one minute does not mean he understands he must "Stay" for 10 minutes. The duration needs to be built up with training.

Distance is where the dog performs the behavior at a distance from the trainer, or the dog stays while the trainer moves around or away from the dog. Avoid working on duration and distance together until a firm foundation has been laid for one or the other.

A Distraction is anything in the environment competing with the animal's attention when being asked to perform a behavior. A handler should start practicing the criterion of distractions in a low distraction area, and then gradually increase the level of distractions.

Teaching the Automatic Sit

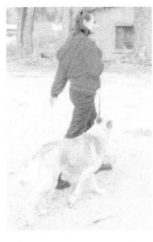

To teach your dog the "Auto-Sit" she must first know how to" Heel".

For the next week, take a walk around your block with your dog. Every few feet and at every curb, stop and have your dog "Sit".

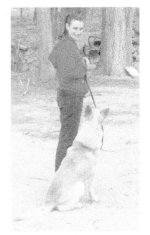

If she knows the command already, tell her to "Sit" verbally. You can also lure her into a "Sit" by using a treat and raising it up and over her head so that she has to look up to see the treat. When she looks up she should fold into a "Sit".

By the end of the week, your dog should be beginning to automatically "Sit" when you come to a halt.

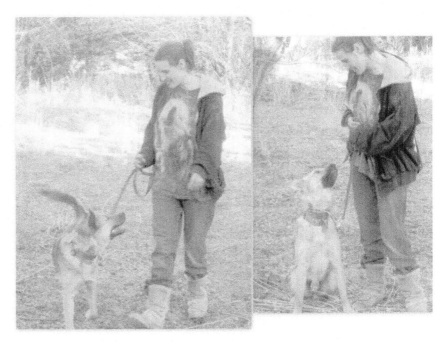

Date:

Training goal of the day:

Lesson Day 17:

Know when to fade the lure.

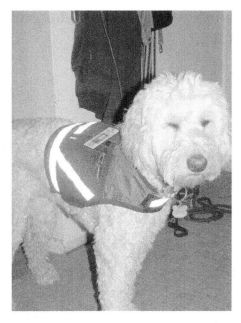

To test the link between a cue and a behavior you have been training, try giving the hand signal or verbal cue without the lure but with your reward marker (clicker).

If the dog follows your cue without luring, begin an intermittent or variable ratio of rewarding. This is also known as "fading the lure".

Now would be a good time to begin "twofers" or rewarding every other time the dog performs the behavior.

The reason it is so critical to begin intermittent reinforcement is that by not doing so leads to sloppy performances or outright refusal from the dog. After all, if she gets a food reward every time, and right now she is not hungry, she knows next time or any time she feels like earning a reward it is always offered, meaning she does not feel motivated to comply with your request right now.

The variable ratio can be compared to different types of machines. A fixed ratio machine, such as a soda machine is expected to give you a beverage when you deposit a certain amount of change. This never changes (well, with the exception of inflation of prices, of course).

A slot game at the casino is on a variable ratio. You never know when it will pay or how much. This variable ratio and feeling the anticipation of not knowing is what keeps people at the machine continuing to put their money in, often until they have no more left. It is pretty safe to say that the anticipation of earning a reward, whether it is at the casino or a food reward to a dog, is often more exciting than actually receiving the reward.

Another tip I would suggest that goes along with this subject is to vary the type of reward you give to your dog so she never knows what she might get, making it even more exciting for her.

Go to your Spot

Your dog's "Spot" or "Place" can be a dog bed, a rug or mat on the floor. Once your dog knows the "Go to your Spot" command, you can take her spot with you anywhere and she will know to lie on it when asked.

** *This command requires your dog knows "Down" as well as a level II or III "Down- stay"*

Step 1-Throw a treat on your dog's "Spot".

Step 2- As she takes notice of this new game, say her name to get her attention and toss the treat in an exaggerated manner to emphasize the motion of what will become the hand signal of pointing at her "Spot" with your index finger.

Step 3- Click and treat even just her front feet touching the "spot" and shape gradually from there.

Step 4- When she gets this step; begin to hold out on rewarding until she has all four paws on the "Spot".

You can go one of two directions at this point as we advance to *Phase II*. You can either finish training that she MUST lie down on her "Spot" or you can finish training that she can be in any position as long as she is on the "Spot" with all four paws.

Most often, the dog will lie down anyway after a couple of minutes if they are consistently trained.

Phase II

I am going to outline insisting that the dog lie down because in my experience, dogs tend to be harder to keep on the spot in early training

81

when they are allowed to stand up.

Step 1- When your dog learns to follow your hand signal (meaning you are on an intermittent schedule of reinforcement and she understands that pointing to the "Spot" means to go there and place all four paws on the "Spot". She also knows that she may or may not get a treat). Begin to cue or lure "Down" and "Stay".

Step 2- Click, treat, release, repeat.

Step 3- Gradually add distance, duration and distractions

Date:

Training Goal of the day:

Lesson Day 18:

Checklist for public access training

Before beginning any public access training, your dog should know the following commands with 90% success rate, both at home and with distractions.

❏ Sit ❏ Down ❏ Stay (sit/down 5 feet away) ❏ Come (Come and sit in front of me) ❏ Heel ❏ Watch Me/Name ❏ Leave-It ❏ Toilet command

• Use lots of treats and praise during public access training. Your dog must learn to focus on you at all times and ignore everything else.

• Always make sure your dog relieves herself prior to entering a store. If your puppy is less than 4 months old and doesn't relieve herself prior to going in a store, do not enter the store in order to minimize the risk of an accident.

• Any time you are out with your dog in uniform you are representing all service dogs. Be respectful of the rights you are given and ensure you and your dog are professional at all times.

The Swing Finish

The "Swing Finish" is a fancy way to get your dog to align himself next to you in the proper "Heel" position from a "Front" position (such as following a recall). After some practice you will be able to cue your dog from anywhere using your index finger as the hand signal. Not only does the "Swing Finish" look impressive, it is very useful as well.

Step 1-With your dog on leash in the front position, hold a treat between your left thumb and second finger. Hold your index finger up to create the hand signal.

Step 2- Slowly move your arm out to the side while taking a couple of steps back and simultaneously luring your dog to walk beside you (your dog is walking forward and you backward).

Step 3- Continue slowly leading your dog to turn a half circle (90 degrees) behind you in order to face the same direction as you are.

Step 4- Both you and the dog will now step forward a couple of steps and come to a halt.

Step 5- Cue or lure "Sit"

Sheena is doing a "Swing Finish". However, she was trained on the right side for her handler.

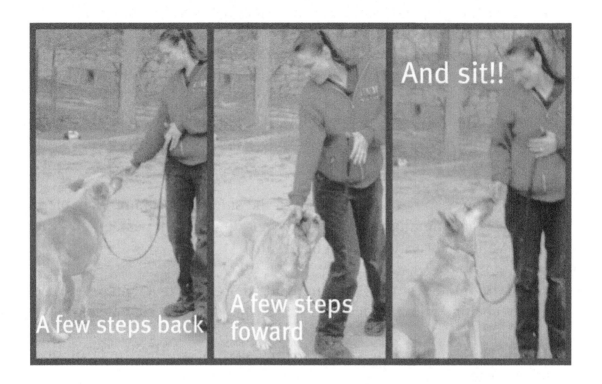

Date:

Training Goal of the day:

Lesson Day 19:

Always end on a positive note

Start your sessions by doing review of something you have already taught and your dog knows. This will build confidence and that helps motivation as well as making training fun for your dog.

During your sessions, introduce new material briefly. If your dog makes progress on the new material, stop there!

Do not be tempted to continue the new material this session. When your dog makes progress and you stop there, this is what she remembers and will be more likely to be successful in future sessions. Also the success builds confidence and we want our dog to have the confidence to try new things while training.

After review and a brief introduction to new material, end the training session on a positive note by doing another review so your dog has another success!

You can add additional motivation to training sessions by offering something valuable to your dog after a session.

**Examples could include a walk, a game your dog enjoys, a car ride, a meal, a few minutes to play with a special toy that your dog enjoys but only gets to play with on certain occasions etc.*

By adding an incentive after training you are rewarding the training and building motivation for future sessions.

Stay Phase II

When your dog will hold a "Stay" reliably without distractions and you within sight for 5 minutes, you can begin *Phase II* by beginning to practice in places with more distractions (a parking lot, the front yard, a quiet area of the park etc.)

Phase II

-Follow the steps from the beginning of *Phase I* in places with more distractions. -Continue practicing at home and begin adding **duration** to the time you ask your dog to "Stay".

-Practice in every room in the house.

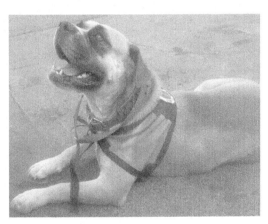

-When you return to your dog to release him, walk around him before you reward and release as a proofing exercise.

Date:

Training Goal of the day:

Lesson Day 20:

Reinforcement strengthens a behavior

Reinforcement, whether positive or negative, strengthens behavior. This is true for all mammals and many other animals as well. In Karen Pryor's book "Don't Shoot the Dog" she gives examples of how to use reinforcement to change behavior.

She does not only give examples pertaining to dogs, however. I think the way she chose to give examples using dogs, cats, roommates, spouses, co-workers etc. is genius! By doing so, she effectively was able to clearly explain how reinforcement and punishment work in a way anyone could understand.

** I highly recommend the book for anyone training a dog or who would like people in their lives to have a shift in certain behaviors as well.

Have you ever thought about how marine mammals or exotic animals are trained? How about animals that do amazing stunts in movies? At the zoo, how do keepers get the tigers, elephants or gorillas to move from one enclosure to another for cleaning?

You cannot put a choke collar on a dolphin and if an elephant does not want to move, it is unlikely a person would be able to move it by force. It would also be potentially dangerous.

The answer to all the above is positive reinforcement, particularly signal or marker training.

TAKE-IT

One of the commands I like to teach service dogs is "Take-it". "Take-it" means to pick up whatever item I specify and hold it or carry it in their mouth. Usually I have them "Bring-it" and then "Give-it".

Keep in mind it will be much easier to teach some dogs than others and much of that depends on the breed of dog. A Retriever may be eager to pick up new items, whereas a Pekingese may be more reluctant.

Method 1

Some dogs will take an object held in front of them but most will need you to get them excited about the object. Pretend it is a toy and wave it around. Say "Are you ready?" and toss the item.

Look for that split second he puts his mouth on it and click, praise and reward. If your dog will not even put his mouth on it, don't worry! Use the clicker and reward any interest he shows in the object.

Gradually you can hold out and ask him for a more precise "Take-it".

Method 2

Method 2 is for dogs that play ball and for dogs who have mastered "Take-it". It can be used in combination with method 1 or alone.

Throw the ball and as your dog picks it up say "Take-it" to label the behavior. When he brings it back say "Drop-it" or "Give-it" as he is doing it. Do not make the mistake of chanting "Take-it" "Take-it "as your dog isn't taking it. Doing so would label the wrong behavior.

Right now as they are learning, we want to label "Take-it" only as the dog is doing it. Later when she knows "Take-it" you can command her to do so.

Make it easy for your dog. Set them up for success. Reward very small increments, especially with dogs that don't readily pick up items in their mouths.

Tip: Most dogs don't like metal in their mouths so consider putting a leather key fob on your keys if you are using them.

Date:

Training Goal of the day:

Lesson Day 21: Be Prepared;
Let's Role Play

What would you say in the following situations? It is a good idea to practice how to talk to the public so that when you are asked awkward questions, you are prepared with an appropriate response.

Always remember that not only are you representing yourself, you are also representing service dogs in general. How you interact with a person will partially determine how they react to those with service dogs in the future.

 - "You don't look like you need a service dog"

-"How did you get that vest? I need to know where to buy one so I can bring my dog into the store"

- "That doesn't look like a service dog

- "I'm allergic to dogs. Please don't bring your dog in here."

- "That dog is a filthy animal. Dogs shouldn't be around when I eat"

- "Your dog shouldn't be doing that. I can tell you how to fix it"

- An Adult starts petting your dog without asking.

What would you say to each comment? What would you do regarding the other situation?

Structured Recall

Phase II

Step 1- Put your dog on a "Stay" (teach Sit and Down separately) Remember to step away from your dog using the foot farthest from him (footwork). Walk out 6 feet or as far as you can without your dog breaking the "Stay". Turn and face your dog.

Step 2- Say your dog's name to get his attention and wait one full second before giving the command.

 **Note: Dogs should NOT anticipate the command and start coming to you when you have only said their name!

Step 3- If the dog holds the "Stay" when you said his name and you have his full attention, give the verbal command and hand signal for "Come". Your dog should be expected to come directly to you, and when he does make a huge fuss and lots of reward and praise.

Step 4- Recalls end with your dog sitting directly in front, facing you. Praise and reward the Recall and the "Sit" separately at first as two different behaviors.

Step 5- Gradually add *distance* as your dog progresses.

Step 6- Repeat 10 times as many times daily as possible.

Date:

Training Goal of the day:

Training Activity:

The Training Game

Object: A game using human subjects to demonstrate what training might feel like to a dog.
Difficulty: Moderate
Prerequisites: Understanding of how the clicker works in training
Items needed: A clicker and at least 2-3 people.

The Training Game was developed by Karen Pryor and used at seminars to show people (who often expect dogs to automatically understand) a different point of view.

One person is chosen to be a trainer and another is the "subject", or in Karen Pryor's case, being a marine mammal trainer, a "dolphin". After the dolphin goes out of earshot, the rest of the group decides what the behavior to be trained will be.

The trainer "trains" the dolphin to perform the behavior using only a nonverbal cue (clicker or other reward marker such as "yes").

You can use a nonsense word if you choose, as long as it gives no clue to the actual behavior chosen to train.

The subject (dolphin) returns to the group and is told only that they are conditioned to a clicker to know that it means they are being rewarded.

I will use an example of a game actually played at one of Karen Pryor's early seminars.

The participants decided to teach the subject to go to the center of the room and spin in a circle.

The subject wanders around the room and receives clicks every time he approaches the center of the room.

The subject starts spending more time in the center and soon only gets clicked when he is actually in the center.

The subject stands in the center, dumbfounded and visibly getting frustrated for a bit. When the subject turns slightly towards the "trainer" perhaps hoping for some sort of visual cue, he earns a click.

The subject goes to the center of the room, does a partial turn and then marches off in another direction. The clicks stop.

Frustrated, the subject goes back to the center and turns towards the trainer. Click!

Subject turns back, nothing. Turns farther and earns a couple of clicks while turning so subject continues turning and eventually spins an entire circle. The group applauds!

Conclusion; once you have had a turn playing the part of the subject, you will certainly have seen a different point of view and most likely will have more compassion and patience while training your dog.

This week I feel proud of my team because:

We need improvement in these areas:

Week 3 Notes:

Lesson Day 22:

Training is a continual process

When you take your dog through obedience training you are advised to practice each command on a daily basis. Many dog owners mistakenly think that they do not have time to work with their dogs every day.

Dogs learn best when they are taught in frequent but short sessions lasting only 10-15 minutes or less. I recommend that my students practice a minimum of three sessions per day. I also recommend that my students look for any opportunity they can to turn an event into a training opportunity.

For example:
-While you are cooking dinner or watching TV why not practice a "Down-stay"?

-Dropped a piece of food on the floor? Practice the "Leave-it" command.

-Dog in the other room? Call her to "Come" and then give lots of praise and a reward when she does.

-Have your dog "Sit" every time he wants something; like a toy, to go out, come in or to go on a car ride.

-Look for a spare five minutes to train anytime you can and incorporate training into your everyday routine whenever possible.

Give-it

"Give-it" is asking your dog to place an item in your hand rather than simply dropping it. I tend to teach "Drop-it" for items your dog is not supposed to have and "Give-it" for items the dog has been asked to retrieve for me.

Step 1- Have a favorite toy or high value treat on hand but out of sight.

Step 2- Have dog pick up a lower value item (or wait until he does).

Step 3- With your higher value item in one hand behind your back, place your other hand under the item in your dog's mouth and present the trade item.

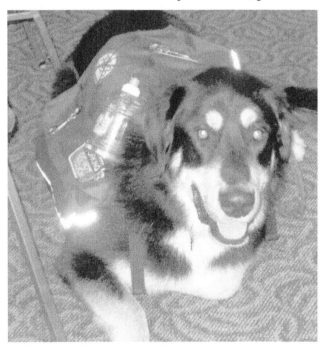

Step 4- As dog drops item in your hand, label the action by saying "Give-it" and give them the trade item.

Date:

Training Goal of the day:

Lesson Day 23:

Life rewards are anything your dog wants, needs or enjoys.

Some examples include:
Going out the door, coming in the door, going for a car ride, going for a walk, receiving affection, mealtimes and the list goes on.

When dogs are handed everything for free, problems can arise. One of any dog's main resources is food. When dogs are given a full bowl of food and allowed to eat at will they tend to take food for granted and many even become picky eaters.

They expect the food to be there and never do they give a thought to where it came from or what they have to do for it. They also never learn to respect the keeper of the food (you) for providing it. Having to work for the food seems to bring more respect for the food and where it comes from. Using mealtimes as a life reward, you can ask your dog to do something in order to earn the reward of enjoying the meal. Even a simple "Sit" will do.

It is important to recognize these ***life rewards*** as things that your dog must always work for and only allow these rewards when your dog has put in the work. Think of it like a paycheck for a job well done. This teaches them to control their impulses and to rely on you to make the reward possible.

Date:

Training Goal of the day:

Lesson Day 24:

Positive reinforcement works on virtually all living beings

Positive reinforcement

Giving of a pleasurable event, increasing the likelihood of a behavior repeating itself in the future.

Positive reinforcement is so simple and effective. It is the absolute foundation of the MEGA LEARNING model of teaching your dog to work with you as a team.

An example of using positive reinforcement in working on a dog's Recall. I chose to give an example of working smarter by using an opportunity to further reinforce the dog's quick response to the Recall.

Here is an example of how the owner could just as easily negatively

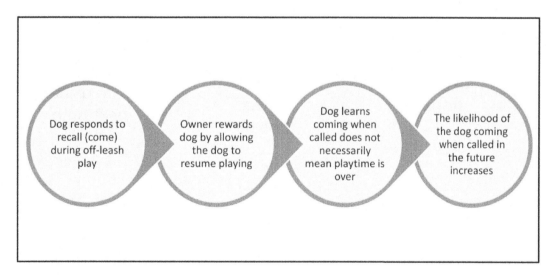

punish the very behavior (prompt Recall) she wants repeated in the future, likely without even realizing it.

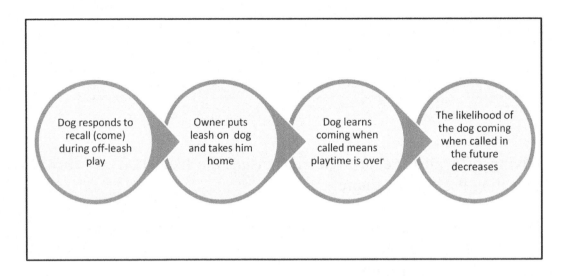

Remember, positive reinforcement can be used with any animal (humans learn by positive reinforcement too).

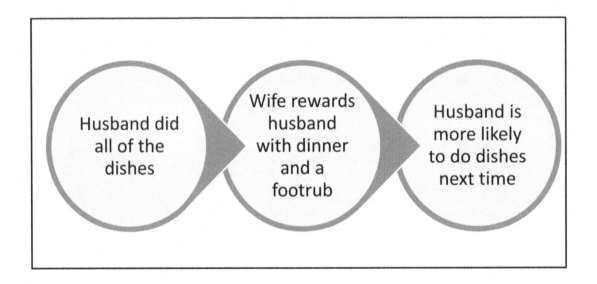

One more thing worth mentioning is that reinforcement and punishment (positive or negative) can come from the environment as well. This is why many of the things dogs do that we would rather they did not do, are self-rewarding by way of the environment being responsible for either reinforcing the behavior or punishing it away.

Take this example of how you or I might be self-rewarded by a choice made.

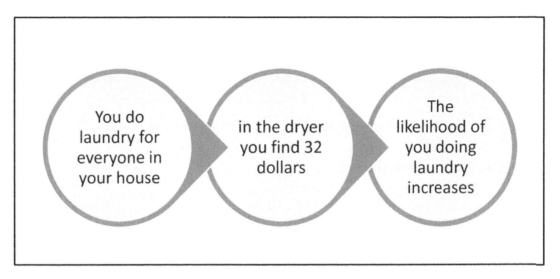

**Positive reinforcement is the foundation for most training programs of any animal, as we have learned. Avoid following advice from a professional who continues to employ outdated methods of traditional training. Ask a professional what methods he or she uses and never follow instruction to use tools that would inflict pain such as a prong collar. It is NOT necessary.*

Under

Step 1-Set a table up in the middle of the room instead of next to a wall with one chair. Sit in the chair with your dog on one side, on-leash.

Step 2- Lure dog under the table using a food reward.

Step 3- Click, treat. release and repeat.

Phase II

Step 1-When dog is comfortable going under table, cue "Down".

Step 2- Click, treat, release and repeat.

Phase III

Step 1- Cue "Under"

Step 2- Cue "Down". And then Cue "Stay".

Step 3-Click, treat, release and repeat.

Date:

Training Goal of the day:

Lesson Day 25:

Negative punishment

Removing of a pleasant event decreasing the likelihood of a behavior repeating itself in the future.

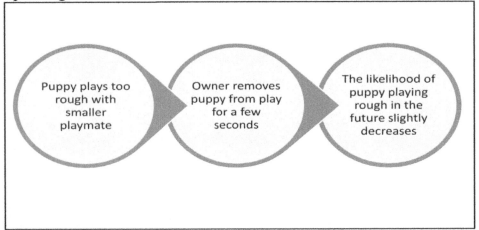

In the above example we see that the consequence is likely effective at helping to decrease the unwanted behavior, in this case a puppy playing too rough.

**If you have trouble with keeping the laws of punishment and reinforcement straight, this may help.*

Reinforcement- Increases **Punishment**-Decreases
Positive- Gives **Negative**-Takes away

Pass

"Pass" is similar to the "Swing Finish", except that the dog follows your right index finger to come from the front of you, along your right side and behind your back to finish by sitting obediently on your left side in the perfect "Heel" position.

Step 1- With your dog on leash in the "Front" position; place a treat between your thumb and second finger on your right hand. Put your index finger up for the hand signal.

Step 2- Extend your arm as you see in the photo and slowly lead your dog using the lure to go along your right side.

Step 3- If possible, pass the treat behind your back (still luring the dog) so he goes behind you and finishes by coming to your left side and facing forward beside you.

Step 4- Cue "Sit"

Step 5- Click and treat

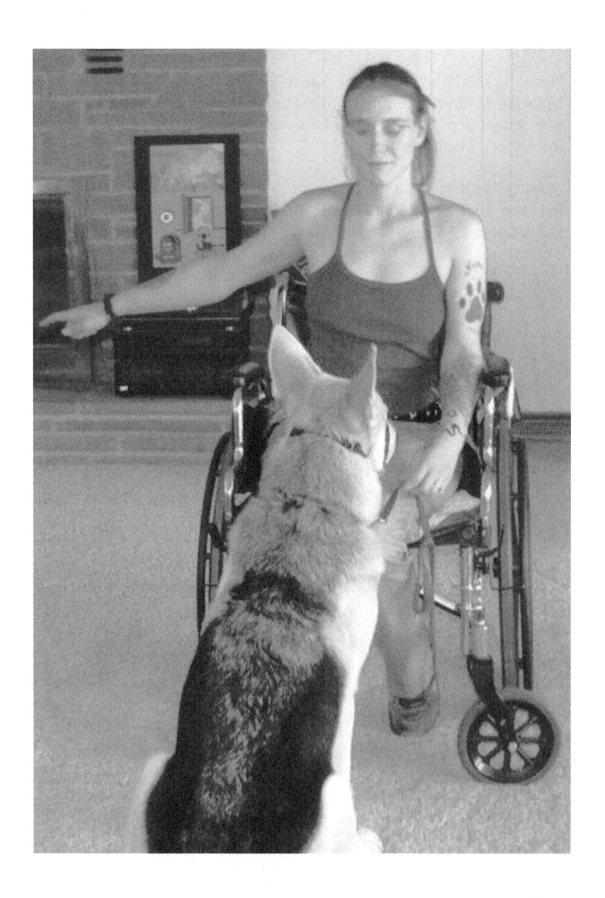

Date:

Training Goal of the day:

Lesson Day 26:

Negative reinforcement can be a great tool

Negative reinforcement

Removal of an unpleasant event increasing the likelihood of a behavior occurring in the future.

Examples: **Please note again, examples of techniques I use do not necessarily reflect methods I use or condone.*

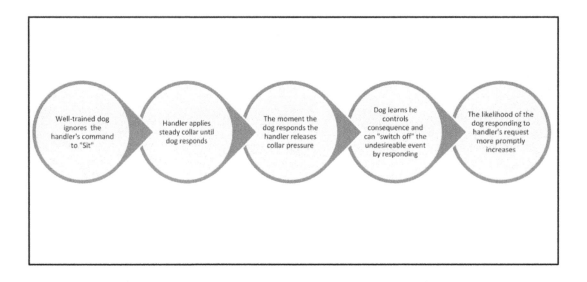

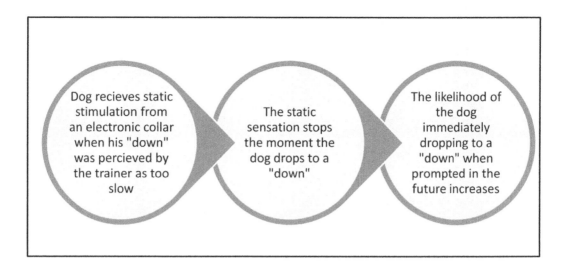

A classic example is B.F. Skinner's "Rat Box".

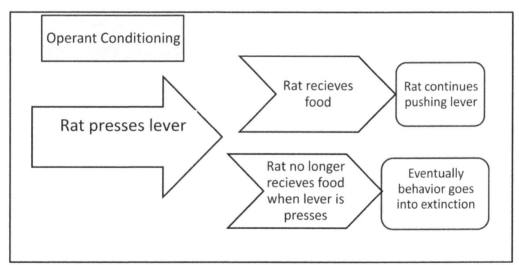

When Skinner added a light that illuminated just prior to the electric shock occurring, the rats learn to push the lever BEFORE the shock occurs.

Date:

Training Goal of the day:

Lesson Day 27:

Positive punishment

Giving of an unpleasant event decreasing the likelihood of a behavior repeating itself in the future.

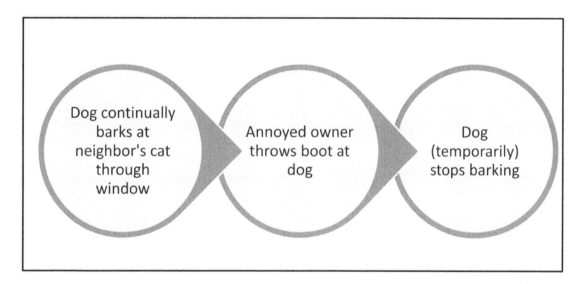

 Above I use an example of positive punishment that demonstrates that in this case this response was effective for the moment. However, do not let the word "positive" confuse you, this is the least effective and yet likely still the most commonly used method of improving your dog's behavior.

Next, I will give another example; this example demonstrates how the owner's use of positive punishment taught the dog nothing since he did not catch the dog offending.

Dog gets into the trash while owner is at work → Annoyed owner swats dog with bits of trash when he gets home → Dog learns nothing about digging in trash

Here I will also add an example from the dog's point of view using the trash raiding incident and focusing on the delayed reprimand:

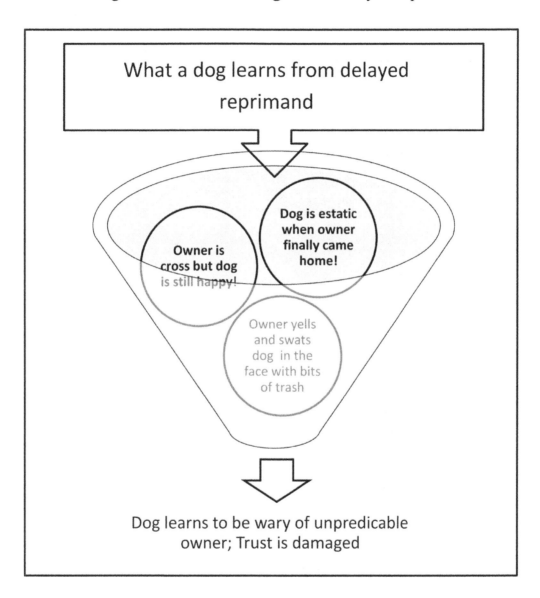

What a dog learns from delayed reprimand

Owner is cross but dog is still happy!

Dog is estatic when owner finally came home!

Owner yells and swats dog in the face with bits of trash

Dog learns to be wary of unpredicable owner; Trust is damaged

Below I list another ridiculous example of "positive" punishment to further stress my point of the inefficiency of positive punishment techniques.

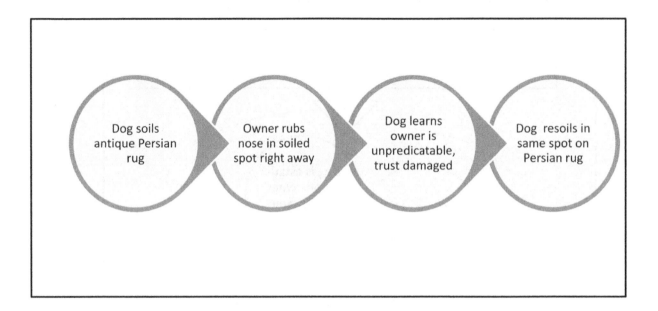

Dog soils antique Persian rug → *Owner rubs nose in soiled spot right away* → *Dog learns owner is unpredicatable, trust damaged* → *Dog resoils in same spot on Persian rug*

**These are not techniques I would use or condone; I am simply offering examples to help explain the concepts.*

Date:

Training Goal of the day:

Lesson Day 28:

The relationship between punishment and negative reinforcement

Punishment and negative reinforcement rarely occur independently. Virtually all aversive training events are a combination of punishment and negative reinforcement.

****For example: A dog is corrected (punished) using a collar correction for straying too far from the "heel" position during an exercise. He is also negatively reinforced once he returns to the "heel" position.*

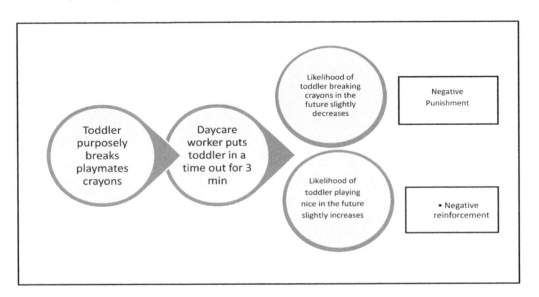

If you look at any punitive event, you will probably find that some behavior is negatively reinforced.

Date:

Training Goal of the day:

Training Activity:

Open and close (French handle) doors, cupboards, drawers, the dryer and the fridge

Difficulty: Moderate
Prerequisite: Tug
Items Needed: Clicker, Treats, Tug toy or Bandana

Open

Step 1: Tie a bandana or rope toy around your door handle. Tell him to "Tug" it. Wait until he tugs the door open, then click and treat.

Step 2: Keep doing this, eventually saying, "Open" whenever he tugs the door open. Click and treat every time.

Step 3: After your training session, he should be able to open the door at your command.

Close

Step 1: Put your target stick or laser pointer light on the door. Your dog can use "Nose" but "Paws" might be better.

Step 2: Each time he touches it and moves the door a little, click and treat.

Step 3: Start waiting until he has pushed the door closed. Click and treat.

Step 4: Do this until he will close the door each time. Click and treat generously when he does this!

Step 5: Start saying "close" when he closes the door. After repeating the action several times, he should close the door at your command.

This week I feel proud of my team because:

We need improvement in these areas:

Week 4 Notes:

This book is dedicated to all of the people I have worked with to help train their own service dogs, those I have placed dogs with for service dog work and to those I have not yet met who are curious and eager to embark on the journey to train their own service dogs.

If you found this workbook helpful, please take a minute and twelve seconds to write a review or even just take thirteen seconds or less to rate it.

Thank you!

Here is a sample schedule that would take 2 weeks to complete the first 7 days in the program

Day 1- Name/Watch me
Day 2- Review 1
Day 3- Review 1, Sit
Day 4- Review 1, 3
Day 5- Review 1, 3, Heel
Day 6- Review 1, 3, 5
Day 7- Review 1, 3, 5, Come; phase I
Day 8- Review 1, 3, 5, 7
Day 9- Review 1, 3, 5, 7, Down
Day 10- Review 1, 3, 5, 7, 9
Day 11- Review 1, 3, 5, 7, 9, Stay; phase I
Day 12- Review 1, 3, 5, 7, 9, 11
Day 13- Review 1, 3, 5, 7, 9, 11, Wait
Day 14- Review 1, 3, 5, 7, 9, 11, 13

Here is another sample schedule to complete the first 7 days over a period of 42 days if that is more your pace:
Day 1- Name/Watch me
Day 2, Day 3, Day 4, Day 5- Review 1
Day 6- Review 1, Sit Day 7, Day 8, Day 9, Day 10- Review 1, 3
Day 11- Review 1, 3, Heel
Day 12, Day 13, Day 14, Day 15- Review 1, 3, 5
Day 16- Review 1, 3, 5, Come; phase I
Day 17, Day 18, Day 19, Day 20- Review 1, 3, 5, 7
Day 21- Review 1, 3, 5, 7, Down
Day 26, Day 27, Day 28, Day 29, Day 30-- Review 1, 3, 5, 7, 9
Day 31- Review 1, 3, 5, 7, 9, Stay; phase I
Day 32, Day 33, Day 34, Day 35, Day 36- Review 1, 3, 5, 7, 9, 11
Day 37- Review 1, 3, 5, 7, 9, 11, Wait
Day 38-43- Review 1, 3, 5, 7, 9, 11, and 13

Final Review

Overall were your training goals from the beginning of the journal met?

What areas still need improvement?

Write each area (If needed) on a separate piece of paper, use what you have learned to create a training plan.

Trained Task # 1

Trained Task # 2

Trained Task # 3

Notes:

Notes:

Notes:

Service Dog Training Log

Date	New Behavior	Review	Achievements	Need to work on

Service Dog Training Log

Date	Notes:

Service Dog Training Log

Date	New Behavior	Review	Achievements	Need to work on

Service Dog Training Log

Date	Notes:

Service Dog Training Log

Date	New Behavior	Review	Achievements	Need to work on

Service Dog Training Log

Date	Notes:

Service Dog Training Log

Date	New Behavior	Review	Achievements	Need to work on

Service Dog Training Log

Date	Notes:

Service Dog Training Log

Date	New Behavior	Review	Achievements	Need to work on

Service Dog Training Log

Date	Notes:						

Service Dog Training Log

Date	New Behavior	Review	Achievements	Need to work on

Service Dog Training Log

Date	Notes:						

Service Dog Training Log

Date	New Behavior	Review	Achievements	Need to work on

Service Dog Training Log

Date	Notes:

About the Author

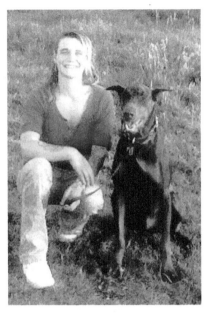

Megan Brooks is a professional dog trainer who has worked with dogs for as long as she can remember. She has specialized in service dog training since 2008.

Megan worked as a Certified Veterinary Technician in the Denver area until she was permanently injured in a motor vehicle accident in 2003.

This is when Megan trained her own dog for mobility assistance and started The Helping Paws Project to help other people with disabilities train their own pets for service dog work.

Megan is a Certified Dog Trainer through the International Association of Canine Professionals (IACP) as well as an AKC Canine Good Citizen Evaluator since 2008.

Megan currently resides in Northern New Mexico where she continues to run the Helping Paws Project & Bulldogs for Soldiers. She also volunteers at the Reuse Center, a recycling/donation facility.

She shares life with 3 Olde English Bulldogges, a Shar-Pei x Pit Bull rescue dog, 2 horses, a cat, a snake and an African Grey Parrot.

Legal Disclaimer

While all attempts have been made to provide the most accurate and current information in this publication, neither the author nor the publisher assume any responsibility or liability whatsoever on the behalf of the purchaser or reader of these materials.

The views expressed are those of the author alone and is for informational purposes only.

The information in this book should never replace the advice you receive from a licensed veterinarian.

.

Made in the USA
Coppell, TX
21 March 2020